The Secrets of Vagus Nerve Stimulation

18 Proven, Science-Backed Exercises and Methods to Activate Your Vagal Tone and Heal from Inflammation, Chronic Stress, Anxiety, Epilepsy, and Depression.

By

Dr. Lee Henton

Copyright © 2020 – Dr. Lee Henton

All rights reserved

No part of this publication may be reproduced, distributed, or transmitted in any form or by any means, including photocopying, recording, or other electronic or mechanical methods, without the prior written permission of the publisher, except in the case of brief quotations embodied in reviews and certain other non-commercial uses permitted by copyright law.

Disclaimer

This publication is designed to provide reliable information on the subject matter only for educational purposes, and it is not intended to provide medical advice for any medical treatment. You should always consult your doctor or physician for guidance before you stop, start, or alter any prescription medications or attempt to implement the methods discussed. This book is published independently by the author and has no affiliation with any brands or products mentioned within it. The author hereby disclaims any responsibility or liability whatsoever that is incurred from the use or application of the contents of this publication by the purchaser or reader. The purchaser or reader is hereby responsible for his or her own actions.

Books By The Same Author

No	Title
A Special Do-It-Yourself Homemade Guide to Protect You From Viruses and Bacteria	
1	The 5-Minutes DIY Homemade Hand Sanitizer
2	The 10 Minutes DIY Homemade Face Mask
3	Homemade Hand Sanitizer and Homemade Face Mask (2 Books In 1)
Other Books Co-written By The Author	
4	The Budget-Friendly Renal Diet Cookbook

Table of Contents

Books By The Same Author 3

About The Author 9

Introduction 10

Chapter 1 17

Getting to Know Your Vagus Nerve 17

What is the Vagus Nerve? 19

Anatomy of the Vagus Nerve 25

    From the Brainstem Connections 26

    Down to the Neck 28

    Down to the Thorax 33

    Down to the Abdomen 34

Why The Vagus Nerve Is So Important 42

    Swallowing of Food 45

    Promotes Digestion 46

    Fights Inflammation 50

    Controls Heart Rate and Blood Pressure 51

    Facilitates Breathing 53

    Provides Ear Sensations 54

    Manages Hunger and Satiety 54

Gut-Brain Communication 57

Chapter 2 61

Vagal Tone and Why It Matters 61

High Vagal Tone – What it Relates to 63

Low Vagal Tone – What it Relates to 64

Measuring Your Vagal Tone 65

    What is Heart Rate Variability? 66

    Checking Your Heart Rate Variability 68

    Interpreting Your Heart Rate Variability Result 72

Increasing Your Vagal Tone 74

Chapter 3 78

Conditions Associated with The Vagus Nerve 78

    Chronic Stress and Anxiety 79

    Trauma, PTSD, and Depression 82

    Lack of Social Interaction 85

    Sleep Disorders and Disruptive Circadian Rhythm 86

    Chronic Inflammation 88

    Dysfunctional Breathing 91

    Dysfunctional Digestive System 94

    Dysfunctional Heart Rate 96

Chapter 4 100

Substances That May Affect Your Vagus Nerve 100

    Botox 100

    Certain Antibiotics 103

    Heavy Metals 106

    Excess Sugar Intake 109

Chapter 5 114

Stimulating Your Vagus Nerve 114

Natural Exercises and Practices 115

    Deep and Slow Breathing 115

    Humming or Chanting 120

    Singing 121

    Humor Therapy 122

    Gargling 123

    Gag Reflex 125

    Exposure to Cold 126

    Sudarshan Kriya Yoga 129

    Loving Kindness Meditation 131

    Exposure to Sunlight 132

    Coffee Enema 134

    Massage 137

    Movement or Exercise 138

Food and Dietary Supplement 140

    Probiotics 140

    Omega-3 Fatty Acids 143

Passive Methods of Stimulation 146

    Auricular Acupuncture 146

Chiropractor Care 148

Electrical Stimulation.. 150

Conclusion 156

References 159

About The Author

Dr. Lee Henton is a US-trained General Practice Doctor from the Johns Hopkins University School of Medicine with additional qualification in nutritional medicine from Iowa State University. He is a certified specialist in dietology and nutrition.

He has extensive years of medical and nutritional experience across general medicine, pediatrics, traumatology, addictions, food nutrition, and diet therapy.

He currently runs a co-established private medical and wellness practice where he operates from. His approach is personalized with each client by combining medical and food nutrition counseling. All advice he provides is at par with his experience, as well as with medical and nutritional concepts. He specializes primarily in men and women's health.

He lives in Minnesota with his wife and two daughters.

Introduction

It is no surprise that most people have not heard of the vagus nerve. With such a name, there is little wonder. Even though the vagus nerve is often overlooked, this nerve plays a significant role in your body and nervous system than you can ever imagine. The vagus nerve is the longest of all the nerves in your body, and it is linked to several parts of your body. It starts in the brain and travels around the body, regulating the control of your digestive system, liver, spleen, pancreas, gallbladder, kidneys, stomach, throat muscles, small intestine, heart, lungs and some part of your large intestine. It works closely with your autonomic nervous system, most especially, your parasympathetic nervous system (what is called your rest and digest state). For instance, the vagus nerve knows when your heart rate increases from an energy-consuming or stressful activity, and immediately, it activates your parasympathetic system which then prepares your body for rest and ensures among others that;

- Your blood pressure is reduced, and all associated conditions such as stroke and heart disease are less likely to occur.

- Your digestive system is more efficient in a way that you don't bloat or become unable to process food.

- Your body produces more enzymes to break down food.

- Your body can regulate blood sugar levels more efficiently that you are at a lower risk of having type 2 diabetes.

- Your body can respond to inflammation, thereby reducing the possibility of related diseases such as IBS, arthritis, lupus, and more.

- Your chance of headaches and migraine are reduced.

- Your mood improves, and
- You feel more relaxed to deal with depression and anxiety.

How well your vagus nerve performs is determinant on the health of your body. The opposite happens when the vagus nerve is not able to support your body and keep you healthy in stressful situations. This would lead to an overactivation of your parasympathetic nervous system, which in turn activates the sympathetic nervous system (fight or flight state) to take over your body. Under consistent and uncontrolled stress levels, our body becomes susceptible to a range of problems such as;

- High blood pressure
- Type -2 diabetes
- Strokes
- Heart disease

- Poor digestion
- Obesity
- Respiratory failure
- Inflammatory disease, such as IBS, arthritis, lupus, etc.
- Depression, and more.

How possible it is you may ask, that these issues which are on the increase in today's modern world, are associated with the malfunctioning of the vagus nerve?

The answer is quite simple. Given that the vagus nerve originates from the brainstem, which is inside your brain and branches out to connect several organs and parts of your body that is responsible for keeping you healthy, any damage to this nerve inadvertently affects the functioning of your organs and your overall health. This damage can be as a result of certain harmful medications used to treat a disease or illness. It could be an injury, an accident, or a surgery that affected this nerve. It could also be the type of food you eat, your kind of lifestyle such as having too much alcohol or excessive smoking, or even something simple as not regularly exercising that could cause damage to this nerve – whichever the case, the result can alter your health and life for the worse. I know this because it happened to me, and I never knew the malfunctioning of this nerve was the cause of my predicament until my quest for a solution led me to a deeper understanding of the vagus nerve and its impact on my health.

Now more than ever, recognizing the role played by your vagus nerve on your overall health and wellbeing is increasingly important and requires that active measures be taken to tend to this nerve.

You don't have to go through what I experienced to understand the importance of this nerve, and why it needs to be cared for. Perhaps you already found yourself in a messy state of health, and you are experiencing one or more of the defects associated with a damaged vagus nerve, you don't have to worry because this book would:

- Enlighten you on several health conditions that is linked to a damaged vagus nerve.

- Describe science-backed exercises and practices, and passive methods of stimulation you can start right away to strengthen your vagus nerve.

- Help you to stimulate and unlock the power of your vagus nerve to heal your body.

- Show you some vital foods and supplements you should take for a healthy vagus nerve.

- Reveal certain substances and lifestyle habits that can damage your vagus nerve and,

- Empower you to take full control of your health and overall wellbeing.

Thank you for downloading this book, I hope you enjoy it!

Chapter 1

Getting to Know Your Vagus Nerve

Picture yourself at home on a Saturday evening after a hectic day. Perhaps to recover from the stress encountered during the day, you decided to give yourself a treat by eating a deliciously cooked meal, and now sitting on your couch to unwind and relax. At this point, you feel wholesomely at rest, so much that you are unaware of how you dozed off so suddenly and falling into a deep sleep. Now while asleep and in your subconscious, you may be thinking your body is as relaxed as you are, whereas a division of your nervous system is actively at work. This division of your nervous system at work, while you are far asleep, is the parasympathetic nervous system, which is busy reducing your heart rate, regulating your breathing, and marching orders to your digestive system organs.

One particular nerve that is heavily involved with the parasympathetic nervous system is the Vagus Nerve (VN).

Our nervous system is made up of about 100 billion nerve cells, which releases information from the brain to the body and vice versa. The vagus nerve is one of the most critical command center responsible for bi-directional communication between the brain and the body. A nerve probably 90% of the population have never heard of or have no clue of its location, nor how powerful this nerve is to the human body. How is it possible that a single nerve that emanates from the brainstem is the longest of all the 12 cranial nerves that connect to the essential organs of the body? Have you ever wondered what could happen to your body should this delicate nerve suffer an injury or gets damaged?

So then, join me and find out.

What is the Vagus Nerve?

Vagus in Latin means "to wander," simply because the vagus nerve wanders from the brain into the body i.e., from the brainstem linking the neck, thorax (chest), and abdomen (belly). The vagus nerve, also referred to as the 10th cranial nerve or cranial nerve X, is not only the longest nerve, but also the most complicated nerve of the 12 pairs of cranial nerves that branches out from the brain.

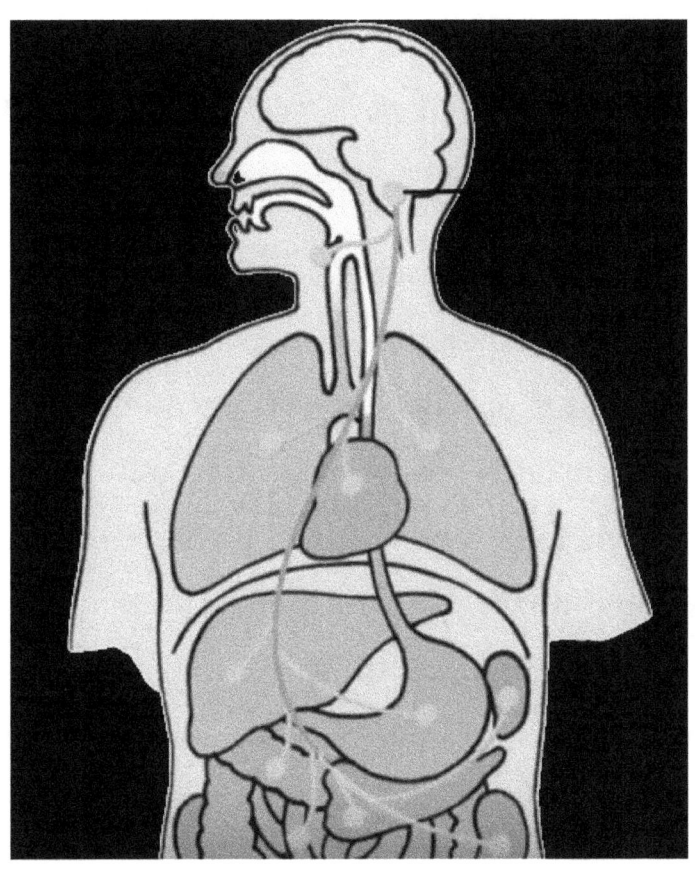

Our body is made up primarily of two nervous systems: the central nervous system and the peripheral nervous system. The latter is further subdivided into the somatic nervous system and the autonomic nervous system. The autonomic nervous system comprises; the sympathetic and the parasympathetic nervous system. The former functions as a "fight or flight" system, just like the gas pedal in an automobile that gears you up to keep firing.

The parasympathetic nervous system, on the other hand, works in the opposite direction. It functions as a "rest and digest" system by slowing you down just like your car brakes – using neurotransmitters such as acetylcholine to reduce your heart rate, blood pressure, and to slow down your organs. The command center for the functioning of the parasympathetic nervous system is your vagus nerve. It is safe to conclude that your vagus nerve is the commander-in-chief when it comes to receiving grace under pressure. It is not the only nerve found in the parasympathetic nervous system, but it is, to a large extent, the most critical nerve since it has the most far-reaching effects on the human body.

Activating the rest and digest state of the parasympathetic nervous system is just one of the many functions performed by the vagus nerve. It is also responsible for facilitating the involuntary (autonomic) activities of the body which includes among others:

- Breathing
- Speech
- Swallowing
- Heartbeat
- Blood Pressure
- Hearing
- Taste
- Blood Circulation
- Digestion
- Bladder Movement
- Sexual Arousal and;

- Gut Health

Although your vagus nerve is the commander-in-chief of receiving grace under pressure, damage to the vagus nerve can cause the parasympathetic response to a fight or flight situation to backfire. For instance, anytime you pull your yourself off a crucial event, feel insecure or intimidated, your vagus nerve would interpret it to mean you are in real danger, thereby exacerbating the situation.

Have you ever asked yourself why you experience the physical symptoms of performance anxiety like a racing heart, sweaty palms, stomach upset, dry mouth, and shaky feeling? These are signs that your vagus nerve is malfunctioning and disengaging. In the absence of a healthy vagus nerve, we only end up having access to parts of our brain that controls primary instincts like fear and fight or flight response.

The healthy functioning of the vagus nerve can be impaired by stress, anxiety, smoking, alcoholism, poor diet, lack of exercise and sleep, or even having part of the nerve accidentally damage during surgery.

When the vagus nerve is not able to perform to the best of its ability, the body and mind become susceptible to a range of conditions which includes but are not limited to:

- Depression
- Anxiety Disorders
- Obesity
- Cardiovascular Disorders
- Hypertension
- Diabetes
- Digestive Disorders

- Chronic Inflammation
- Kidney Malfunction and;
- Parkinson's Disease

Luckily, you can harness the power of your vagus nerve and keep it engaged to release grace when under pressure. When you understand the incredible power your vagus nerve has, you would be geared not only to start practicing ways to exercise its strength to keep you at rest when in distress but also to keep you healthy – physically and mentally.

Anatomy of the Vagus Nerve

As much as possible without being very technical, I would explain the origin of the vagus nerve, and its structural form as it travels all the way through to the organs where it innervates and sends information to and from the brain.

From the Brainstem Connections

The neurons that give rise to the vagus nerve starts in the brainstem, which stems from four nuclei – the dorsal motor nucleus, ambiguous nucleus, solitary nucleus, and spinal trigeminal nucleus. Each of one these exercise control over certain fibers of the nerve. The sensory neurons retrieve signals directly from the skin, which the vagus nerve innervates to the spinal trigeminal nucleus (it includes a certain part of the ear skin, which plays an important role when the vagus nerve is activated using acupuncture treatment). The vagus nerve brings the signals from the internal organs to the solitary nucleus, which are then taken to the brain for further processing. Examples of these signals are those from the stomach, lungs, heart, intestinal tract, gall bladder, liver, spleen, and pancreas. Our body can also pass direct signals to these organs via the vagus nerve by the parasympathetic fibers – originating from the dorsal motor nucleus. These signals are necessary because they provide support in calming and regulating the function of the heart and lungs, while also increasing the actions of the gut and intestinal tract, pancreas, liver, spleen, and gallbladder.

Neurons that perform a motor function, especially to control most of the muscles (the muscles which ensure the airway is kept open, as well as producing sound using the vocal cords) found in the throat and upper airway, are sent out by the nuclei called nucleus ambiguous.

It is important to note that the only nerves in the human body with four separate functions and separate nuclei that contributes to the component fibers are the right and left vagus. On the other hand, the majority of the other nerves found in the human body carry simple sensory information from the skin to the muscles. This differentiation only goes to show how vital the vagus nerve truly is and how extensive its functions are in the human body.

Having looked at the vagus nerve from the brainstem, let's replicate same for the neck, thorax (chest area), and abdomen (belly or tummy area).

Down to the Neck

Right from the medulla oblongata (resident in the brainstem), fibers of the left and right vagus nerves extend directly to the cranial cavity (the inside of the skull), converging to form what is called the vagus nerve – this then passes out of the skull via an opening (the jugular foramen). This jugular foramen is a vast space between the neck and the skull that provides room for the vagus nerve and other blood vessels to pass through. Once the vagus nerve exits the skull, it then enters the upper neck just behind the ear, which sits in-between two blood vessels i.e., the internal carotid artery and the internal jugular vein – our blood's direct lines to and from the brain. The location of the vagus nerve just close to these two blood vessels goes to show how critical this 10th cranial nerve is. Damage of this nerve would most certainly lead to inadequate functioning of most organs of the body, while damage to the blood vessels can result in an outright death. Just after the vagus passes the jugular foramen, exists a thickening of the vagus nerve referred to as the superior ganglion (or jugular ganglion) – a nerve's thickening, formed by a group of sensory neuron cell bodies very close to each other. These cell bodies congregate inside the ganglion, reforming into the thinner nerve section, thereby paving the way for the first branch of the vagus nerve called the auricular branch.

The auricular branch goes back into the skull via the mastoid canaliculus (an opening) toward the ear via another opening of the skull, the tympanomastoid fissure. The auricular branch is sensitive to touch, wetness, and temperature felt on the skin of the ear most especially, the external canal, auricle, and tragus – the major target for activating the treatment of the VN dysfunction with the aid of auricular acupuncture (acupuncture is directed to the ear, and is discussed in more details later in this book).

Just as the vagus nerve starts to pass downward from the superior ganglion, the VN thickens once more, giving rise to the inferior ganglion (also referred to as the nodose ganglion) – which houses the cell bodies of the neurons involved in retrieving information from the internal organs. The vagus nerve again thins out and instantly goes into a passageway made by the carotid sheath (a thickening of connective tissue). In the carotid sheath, the vagus nerve goes into its next branch called the pharyngeal branch. Although this branch has neurons that come directly from the vagus nerve, it also provides some supporting neurons from the ninth and eleventh cranial nerves. As soon as these neurons meet, they will go through the midline of the body until they get to the upper part of the throat (the pharynx). In the pharynx, motor signals are sent to several muscles by the vagus nerve. These muscles play a role in swallowing, in the opening and closing of the upper airway, as well as in the maintenance of the gag reflex. The vagus nerve goes into its third branch (the superior laryngeal nerve) as it travels down the sides of the neck. Immediately, the superior laryngeal nerve branches from the VN after the pharyngeal branch, providing motor signals to the muscles of the larynx. These muscles are responsible for controlling your voice's pitch. As the VN further goes down via the carotid sheath, the cervical cardiac branches arise – the two of three branches innervating the heart, while the third branch (thoracic cardiac branch) appears just after exiting the carotid sheath in the thorax (chest).

These branches interrelate with the nerves of the sympathetic nervous system and form the cardiac plexus (plexi as its plural form). Plexi is made up of a collection of intermingling nerve fibers of several branches and several origin nerves that traverses toward a targeted area). There are two cardiac plexi – the superficial cardiac plexus, located in front of the aorta, and the deep cardiac plexus, located at the back of the aorta (aorta is the main blood vessel that transports blood from the heart to other parts of the human body). At this point, one vital thing to take note of is that the fibers of the cardiac plexi control the rate of the electrical activity responsible for pumping your heart.

Down to the Thorax

Upon exiting the carotid sheath, the vagus nerve goes right down into the thorax, specifically at the back of the first and second ribs, as well as in the front of the wider blood vessels extending from the heart. The left vagus nerve goes in front of the aorta (at the arch), which then gives rise to its fourth branch (the left side recurrent laryngeal nerve). Right across the other side of the body, the right vagus nerve takes a similar route, but instead, it goes in front of the right subclavian artery, sending off its fourth branch (the right side recurrent laryngeal nerve). These branches convey motor signals directly from the brainstem to the muscles of the larynx, which are vital to produce your vocal sounds. Once the vagus nerves get to where the aorta is, the left and right of its nerves sendoff branches to the pair of lungs. A pulmonary branch channeled to the anterior pulmonary plexus is sent by the left vagus nerve, while a pulmonary branch channeled to the posterior pulmonary plexus is sent by the right vagus nerve. The nerve branches mingle with sympathetic neurons, regroups, and after that, travels to innervate the lungs on each side. Based on what the body needs, these branches would navigate its way to the bronchi and the broader branches of the lungs, opening and closing them accordingly.

Down to the Abdomen

The organs of the abdomen are the last section that the vagus nerve innervates. These organs are very critical to the human body because it aids digestion, controls the immune system, and prevents the blood supplied to our cells from having any form of toxins that could affect the health of our cells.

The stomach is the first branch of the abdomen where the vagus nerve goes. The muscles of the stomach are stimulated to function by the vagus nerve fibers when the body is in the rest and digest state. Signals are sent to the parietal cells by the vagus nerve to secrete hydrochloric acid, to the chief cells to secrete digestive enzymes (pepsin and gastrin), and to the stomach's muscle cells to churn and push the food in the stomach into the small intestine. If there is damage to the vagus nerve and these vital signals to the stomach's cells are not being sent, problems such as hypochlorhydria, or what is called low stomach acid will arise – a major root cause of several health issues.

The liver is the second branch of the abdomen, where the vagus nerve goes. These branches are responsible for the sensations you feel when hungry. The food we eat first goes to the stomach where it is broken down, and from there, it goes to the small intestine, where the majority of our macronutrients such as fats, amino acids, and carbohydrates are absorbed into the bloodstream. These nutrients then travel into the liver where they are filtered, processed, and prepared for transporting signals back to the brain. From the liver, information is relayed to the brain by the vagus nerve concerning blood sugar balance, fat intake, as well as the general functioning of the liver. Information concerning the amount of bile required to aid in the digestion of fats can also be relayed to the brain. The liver performs several functions that require the input of the vagus nerve, which includes but not limited to the production of bile and bile salts; production of glucose for balancing the blood sugar; and managing hunger and satiety. Generally speaking, the liver is very vital to our overall wellbeing. However, the innervation of the vagus nerve plays a major role in keeping this balance. The gallbladder, which is closely linked with the liver is very vital for the maximum functioning of our bodies. When our liver creates what is known as bile and bile salts, they are then transported to the gallbladder, where they are stored in preparation for our next meal. As soon as we start our next meal, bile is then pumped by the gallbladder into the first part of the small intestine (the duodenum), which helps to transport fats into the bloodstream. The vagus nerve, yet again, is responsible for mediating the pumping by the gallbladder. From the liver, the vagus never courses to send signals to the gallbladder, and in the process, it activates the muscle cells in its walls, which then pumps bile into the digestive tract.

The pancreas being the next branch of the vagus nerve, is one of the most vital glands in our body, having both an endocrine and exocrine component. The endocrine part of the pancreas secretes insulin and glucagon into the bloodstream, which helps to balance the level of glucose in the blood. The exocrine component of the pancreas, on the other hand, secretes digestive enzymes via a duct into the small intestine. These digestive enzymes are protease (which breaks down proteins into amino acids), lipase (which breaks down fats into fatty acids and cholesterol), and amylase (which breaks down carbohydrates into sugars). The innervation of the vagus nerve transports signals from the pancreas to the brainstem, in which information about the cell status of the endocrine and exocrine are relayed. Information that pertains to the intake of food, as well as the enzymes required to be produced and released into the bloodstream and digestive tract, are also relayed from the brainstem to the organ – the innervation of the vagus nerve is vital for transmitting this information. As soon as the vagus nerve travels past the stomach, the celiac plexus is then formed (a network that exists between the lumbar sympathetic nerves and the parasympathetic fibers of the vagus nerve). This network sends branches to the other parts of the organs in the abdomen. The spleen is the first organ that is innervated after the celiac plexus. The location of the spleen can be traced to the left side of your body, below your left lung, which is opposite your liver. The spleen is responsible for monitoring the bloodstream, as well as the activation or deactivation of the cells of the immune system based on the senses it receives. The sympathetic branch of the nervous system sends information to the spleen to activate the inflammatory pathways, turning on responses to any physical and biochemical trauma or damage. On the other hand, the parasympathetic branch of the nervous system sends information to the spleen to halt the inflammation processes – an area where the vagus nerve is also actively involved.

After the celiac plexus, the next branch of the vagus nerve courses to the small intestine. As soon as the food is churned in the stomach by chemical and physical processes, it then travels to the small intestine where the pancreatic digestive enzymes and bile further process it. The small intestine functions by breaking down and absorbing most of our body's macronutrients, which include fats, proteins, and carbohydrates. The macronutrients which the lining cells of the small intestine have accepted are also received by the bloodstream. When we take in bites of food (called chyme in the digestive process), it is pushed down the length of the small intestine. For this to occur, the muscle cells of the digestive tract are first activated by the vagus nerve by sending signals to the network of nerves lining the gut – these networks of nerves lining the gut are referred to as the enteric nervous system. The bacteria in our body have a significant relationship with the rest of the cells that live in our digestive tracts, i.e., the symbiotic relationship of our human cells with the bacteria in our gut (the microbiome). Although most of our bacteria allies (which produces vital minerals, vitamins, and biochemical for us) are housed in the large intestine of the digestive tract, they can also generate several toxins and gas. The vagus nerve provides a relay path where the microbiome can communicate with our brain, which is very necessary to keep these bacteria in check, by signaling our brain on the functional status of the digestive tract and the microbiome. Approximately in the first half of the large intestine (the ascension and traverse colon) is where the vagus nerve innervates.

The last organ the vagus nerve innervates is the kidney. The function of the kidney (each located on the sides of the body) is to filter out fluid called urine – the blood pressure is a significant determinant of this control. The vagus nerve, which plays a significant role in controlling the function of the kidney, also plays a very vital role in managing the blood pressure. The vagus nerve does not just end at its course; instead, it gives rise to the last plexus with the parasympathetic nerve fibers that courses from the spinal cord's lower end. These fibers are what innervates the other half of the large intestine, which are the descending and sigmoid colon, the bladder, and the sex organs.

Why The Vagus Nerve Is So Important

The vagus nerve is one of the most vital nerves of the human body because it connects not only multiple organs, but also facilitates several processes that take place in our body by actively providing support to the workings of the autonomic nervous system. If you carefully followed me as I took on the anatomy of the vagus nerve in the previous section, you should have picked up several functions performed by this nerve.

Generally, the function of the vagus nerve is broken into four main parts:

Sensory

The sensory function of the vagus nerve is divided into two components, with each performing two different roles:

Somatic Component—This provides somatic sensations for the skin (i.e., sensations behind the ear or the outside area of the ear canal), as well as some regions of the throat.

Visceral Component—This provides visceral sensations experienced in the organs of the body (i.e., sensations for the heart, lungs, larynx, heart, esophagus, trachea, as well as a majority of the digestive tract).

Special Sensory

The vagus nerve plays a minor role in the taste sensation (i.e., taste sensation provided to the root of the tongue).

Motor

The motor function of the vagus nerve stimulates the muscles (responsible for swallowing and speech) in the pharynx, larynx, and the soft palate.

Parasympathetic

The parasympathetic function of the vagus nerve;

- Stimulates the muscles in the heart by regulating the heart rhythm

- Stimulates the muscles in the digestive tract to contract— which includes the stomach, esophagus, and most of the intestines, thereby paving the way for food to navigate through the tract.

Although the vagus nerve function is made up of four main parts, which I summarily touched on, I would go a little deeper into some of these functions.

Swallowing of Food

Whether you agree or not, swallowing is one of the most complex activity your body performs. This is true since it involves some intricate coordination between your brain and some specific nerves and muscles. For food swallowing to occur, the coordination of these muscles, pharynx (throat), larynx (voice box), and esophagus (the hollow tube that transports food from your throat to your stomach) is required. These muscles are all controlled by the cranial nerves, prominent amongst them is the vagus nerve – which allows for the swallowing of each bite of food by pausing the breathing reflex to prevent you from choking. The pharyngeal branch, as earlier discussed, is the second branch of the vagus nerve that manages the muscles of the pharynx. These muscles are the three constrictor muscles located behind the throat and the other two muscles that connects the throat to the soft palate (soft tissue behind the roof of the mouth). These muscles play a vital role in the pharyngeal phase of swallowing by pushing your chewed food down to the larynx as well as to the esophagus while keeping it away from the trachea, thereby ensuring your airway is cleared from food particles.

Promotes Digestion

The vagus nerve plays a significant role in managing the complex processes of your digestive system, which includes sending signals to the muscles of your stomach to contract and to push down the food into the small intestine. Your digestive system, in simple terms, relies on the vagus nerve to function correctly.

Let me give you a quick rundown of how the vagus nerve aids digestion beginning from your stomach all through to your intestines.

Stomach

Once the food swallowing process is completed and the food is pushed down your stomach, your vagus nerve would trigger the production of a certain amount of acid (gastric or stomach acid) in your stomach that helps to properly digest your food, kill bacteria, and absorb specific nutrient such as protein.

Pyloric Sphincter

The pyloric sphincter sits at the base of your stomach, allowing food (chyme) to exit the stomach into the intestines. The vagus nerve is responsible for triggering the opening and closing of the pyloric sphincter – this is to ensure that the food does not stay in the stomach any longer than is necessary.

Gallbladder

The gallbladder, which connects to the bile duct of the liver, receives and stores bile, which, when released, helps with the proper digestion of fats contained in the food (chyme). The vagus nerve is responsible for stimulating the release of bile to the gall bladder and having both direct and indirect control over the functioning of the gall bladder.

Pancreas

The pancreas secretes digestive enzymes that help to digest and absorb nutrients in food, most importantly, fats, and proteins. Partial regulation of the pancreatic functions is achieved when the parasympathetic fiber innervates the pancreas (originating in the dorsal motor nucleus of the brain). This regulation is made possible by the vagus nerve, which also exercises direct control over the secretion of digestive enzymes.

Sphincter of Oddi

Sphincter of Oddi is a muscular valve that exercises control over the flow of bile and pancreatic enzymes into the small intestine. The vagus nerve stimulates the opening of the sphincter of Oddi to allow the flow of bile and pancreatic enzymes from the gallbladder and pancreas into the small intestine.

Intestines
Once the food (chyme) gets to the small and large intestine respectively, the vagus nerve would then stimulate the mixing and shifting of chyme, back and forth, allowing the proper absorption of nutrients into the bloodstream – this process is called peristalsis.

Without the proper functioning of the vagus nerve, proper peristalsis would not occur, which can lead to gastroparesis, bloating, constipation, and discomfort. If partially digested food remains in your intestines without being moved around, your body will absorb the toxins and free radicals that are produced, resulting in a potential chronic inflammation of the intestinal tract.

Fights Inflammation

The vagus nerve plays a vital role in fighting inflammation. A given amount of inflammation after an injury or infection is not out of place – this is the way our body notifies the immune system to heal and repair damaged tissue to protect our body against viruses and bacteria. However, if left uncontrolled and it gets out of hand, it could become chronic, leading to several autoimmune diseases such as rheumatoid arthritis and lupus. The vagus nerve is like a vast network of nerve fibers, positioned all around your organs like spies. When it receives the pro-inflammatory cytokine signal (substances the inflammatory cells secrete, affecting other cells) or a substance called tumor necrosis factor (TNF), it sends an alert to the brain to produce anti-inflammatory neurotransmitters which then regulate the body's immune response accordingly, thereby helping to manage stress and improving how the body responds to pain and illness.

Controls Heart Rate and Blood Pressure

The vagus nerve controls the heart rate and blood pressure through electrical impulses to the heart's natural pacemaker, the sinoatrial node (a group of cells in the wall of the heart's right atrium), where a neurotransmitter called acetylcholine is released to slow the pulse rate and blood pressure if it's too high, keeping a constant rhythm of the heart and thereby preventing tachycardia - a condition that causes your heart to beat more than 100 times per minute. By measuring the time interval between consecutive heartbeats over a given period of time, your heart rate variability (HRV) can be determined. The HRV data can provide valuable insights about the strength of your vagus nerve and the resilience of your heart.

Many studies have been reported on the benefits of stimulating the vagus nerve in patients with heart failure. A study conducted in 2011, as published in the European Heart Journal, reported that continuous stimulation of the vagus nerve could improve the efficiency of the heart to pump blood in patients suffering from heart failure. Similar results were reported in 2014 as published in the journal of cardiac failure where after six months of stimulating the vagus nerve of patients with heart failure, their heart pumped 4.5% more blood per beat than it did prior to the stimulation. More on the methods of vagus stimulation are covered in later sections of this book.

Facilitates Breathing

The vagus nerve pays close attention to how you breathe and sends a signal to the brain and heart to respond accordingly. When you breathe slowly, the oxygen demand of the heart muscle (myocardium) drops, and your heart rate reduces. In stressful situations, taking a slow deep breath would stimulate the vagus nerve to calm you down. If the vagus nerve does not stimulate the release of acetylcholine to the brain, your brain would be unable to communicate with your diaphragm (muscles at the base of your chest which contracts and forces your lungs to expand and take in air), and you won't be able to breath – this would essentially lead to death so to speak. This is why exposing your body to Botox, and mercury most especially can potentially cause severe damage to your vagus nerve, because it interrupts the production of acetylcholine.

Provides Ear Sensations

As earlier discussed in the anatomy of the vagus nerve, the auricular branch (the first branch of the vagus nerve), helps in providing sensations such as touch, wetness, and temperature to certain areas of the ear (e.g., the external canal, auricle, and tragus areas). This is very important because sensations of the ear can be stimulated by the vagus nerve when the auricular acupuncture method of stimulation is used.

Manages Hunger and Satiety

Has it ever crossed your mind why some people get full so easily after eating a small amount of food, and other people still feel hungry not until they have eaten a large amount of food? This is your vagus nerve at work.

The vagus nerve, as we know, connects your gut to your brain, and one type of signal that travels up and down the vagus nerve via this connection is the hunger and satiety signal.

This is how it works...

In the course of eating a meal, the quantity of food present in your stomach stimulates the vagus nerve to send satiety signals to your brain. Your brain then flips by saying, "full." This is how you stop feeling hungry after a meal.

Your gut contains several nutrient-sensing receptors that recognize when you have gotten enough of certain nutrients such as carbohydrates, proteins, and fats. These nutrient-sensing receptors include serotonin, ghrelin, and gustducin. These receptors may or may not be activated, which depends on whether the food you eat contains those nutrients. Vagus nerve is the means by which your brain receives the hunger or satiety nutrient signal. However, when the vagus nerve is damaged and underperforms, those vital satiety signals from your stomach and the intestines would not be able to travel back to your brain. The implication of this is that you would more than likely exhibit a continuous feeling of hunger, lack of satiety, and end up overeating in the process.

Let me paint a clearer picture of what I am trying to communicate...

Remember the nutrient receptors I mentioned earlier? One of such receptors that sense glucose is gustducin (a glucose taste receptor in your gut). A damaged vagus nerve can prevent this receptor from sending signals to the brain that you've had enough sugars and carbs, which could essentially lead to an overdose of glucose, impaired insulin secretion, and potentially resulting in obesity if the situation remains uncontrolled.

Gut-Brain Communication

Does going with your "gut feelings" to make a decision sounds familiar to you? Or have you ever felt "butterflies in your stomach" when you are nervous? If you have experienced any of these, then you are most likely receiving signals from the *second* brain (enteric nervous system) in your gut (specifically, your stomach and intestines).

Your "gut feelings" so to speak are signaled to the brain via the vagus nerve through electrical impulses. It is often said that the vagus nerve cells are 80% afferent, meaning your brain receives more signals from your body while only 20% are efferent, i.e., your brain sends fewer signals to your body – the reason why the term body-mind connection is often used.

In your gut lies what is called the microbiome (tens of trillions of bacteria composition and other microorganisms). These microbiomes play a very important role by enabling the release of critical neurotransmitters such as Serotonin, GABA, and Dopamine that regulates your mood, thinking capabilities, and memory, among many others. So, for instance, whenever you experience any emotions or sensations in your body, be it a broken heart, anger, sadness, anxiety, or happiness, your gut microbiome is more than likely the reason for this. You experience these emotions because these neurotransmitters in your body have sent signals to your brain through your vagus nerve. This communication system between your gut and your brain is what is referred to as the gut-brain axis.

The feedback loop between the gut, vagus nerve, and the brain goes beyond our emotions or sensations. Several other signals are sent along this axis. The goings-on in our guts can, as a matter of fact, be a life or death situation. If the gut is empty, the vagus nerve must inform the brain; if the gut has a problem that will hinder the processing of food and nutrition absorption, the brain must be notified; if the gut is being attacked by pathogens, the brain needs to be in the loop – with status report being constantly updated between the gut and brain.

Think of the vagus nerve as that superhighway communication that ensures your body is in constant touch with your brain. Given that the vagus nerve operates in tandem with the gut microbiome to facilitate the gut-brain communication, it has become increasingly important to not only take proper care of your vagus nerve but also your gut health by engaging in gut-friendly practices such as:

- Taking probiotic supplements or eating fermented foods rich in probiotics such as yogurt, kefir, sauerkraut, cheese, kimchi, sauerkraut, kombucha, and miso

- Avoiding the use of certain antibiotics
- Less consumption of sugary foods and artificial sweeteners
- Regular exercise
- Getting enough sleep
- Cutting down on diets with animal fat
- Eating foods with omega-3 fats and;
- Eating more prebiotic-fiber foods such as asparagus, bananas, chicory, garlic, Jerusalem artichoke, onions, and whole grains.

Note: Some of the above are covered in detail toward the tail end of this book.

Chapter 2

Vagal Tone and Why It Matters

The vagus nerve activity of some people is healthier and stronger than others, which allows their bodies to quickly relax after a stressful activity.

For example, the stress you go through when you subject your body to a high degree of exercise is good, especially when you are done with the exercise, and your body gains health and strength – giving you a positive mental feeling of your achievement. Another example is the positive feeling you get when you complete a stressful task, the feeling of "yes, I did it!". This feeling of accomplishment will gear you up as you prepare for subsequent stressful assignments knowing that you have the situation under control.

The point I am passing across is that a repetitive positive fight or flight response is good if a positive emotion is associated with the completion of the stressful event. Nonetheless, continuous fight or flight response becomes unhealthy if no positive result is associated with the event. Examples of such event are found in our everyday life which includes work, school, finance, and family – falling short in these areas could easily run us down. The impact of this would result in a low vagal tone, which, if sustained for an extended period of time, may lead to poor health and performance.

Please bear in mind that other factors can also cause a low vagal tone, such as poor lifestyle habits, while vagus-friendly habits can increase your vagal tone. In other words, the strength of your vagus response or the degree to which your vagus nerve is active is known as your vagal tone.

It is also interesting to know that based on studies carried out in this area, vagal tone is passed on from mother to child. The implication is that mothers who experience depression, anxiety, or feel angry during their pregnancy have lower vagal activity. And as soon as their child is birthed, the newborn would also have low vagal activity coupled with low dopamine and serotonin levels.

High Vagal Tone – What it Relates to

How strong your vagal tone is would determine how strong your body would function. A high vagal tone would improve your body systems, such as regulating your blood sugar levels, reducing the risk of diabetes, stroke, cardiovascular disease, and migraines, and improving your digestion, among others. A high vagal tone is also associated with better mood, more resilience to stress, and less anxiety. A vagal tone that is high is a pointer to a high heart rate variability (more on this is discussed in the subsequent section).

Low Vagal Tone – What it Relates to

Having a low vagal tone simply means the strength of your vagus nerve response is low. Having a low vagus response could lead to several health conditions such as cardiovascular diseases, strokes, diabetes, depression, negative moods, chronic fatigue, and a higher chance of being affected by inflammations such as autoimmune diseases (rheumatoid arthritis, inflammatory bowel disease, and more). A low vagal tone points to a low heart rate variability.

For instance, a study shows that people with inflammatory conditions most times have low heart rate variability, which can trigger the release of pro-inflammatory cytokines, leading to increased sympathetic nervous system activity and stress hormones.

Measuring Your Vagal Tone

Vagal tone is measured when you track your heart rate alongside your breathing rate. Your heart rate increases when you breathe in and decreases when you breathe out. The difference between the heart rate inhalation and heart rate exhalation is your vagal tone. This difference by the standard is called the heart rate variability. Consequently, to determine if your vagal tone is either low or high, you first have to measure the variation of time (in milliseconds) between consecutive heartbeats, called the heart rate variability (HRV) – a golden standard in measuring the strength of the vagal tone.

What is Heart Rate Variability?

Heart rate variability can be traced to our autonomic nervous system, divided into the sympathetic (fight or flight) and the parasympathetic (rest and digest) nervous system, and is responsible for regulating important body systems such as our heart rate, breathing, blood pressure, and digestion. Heart rate variability is a pointer that both nervous systems are functioning.

Intrinsic heart rate is the measurement of a condition where there is no regulation by neither the parasympathetic nor sympathetic nervous system. When the intrinsic heart rate is prevented from autonomic regulation, a healthy heart contracts within the range of 60-100 beats per minute.

Regulation by the parasympathetic nervous system reduces your heart rate from the intrinsic level while providing variability between successive heartbeats. Parasympathetic regulation almost instantly affects a change on a few heartbeats at a time, after which the heart rate reverts to the intrinsic rate. Sympathetic regulation, on the other hand, increases your heart rate from the intrinsic rate, with little or no room for variability between successive heartbeats. Several consecutive heartbeats are affected by the regulation of the sympathetic nervous system.

The implication of this is that when a person is in the rest and digest response state, the heart rate would be lower but with a higher HRV while in a fight or flight response state, the heart rate would be higher but with a lower HRV.

Factors such as stress can cause the parasympathetic nervous system to be deactivated while activating the sympathetic nervous system even when you are resting.

Research over the years shows that people with a high HRV would exhibit greater cardiovascular fitness and with higher resilience to stress, while people with low HRV would manifest conditions such as depression, anxiety, and cardiovascular disease.

In general, HRV can provide you with feedback on your lifestyle, which can be a great way to determine how your nervous system is not only responding to the environment but also to your feelings, thoughts, and emotions.

Checking Your Heart Rate Variability

Healthy irregularities accompany a healthy heartbeat. Let's say your heart rate is 60 beats per minute; this does not imply your heart beats once in every second. A variation exists among the intervals between your heartbeats. For example, the interval between your successive heartbeats may be 0.5 ms between two consecutive beats and 1.5 ms between another two consecutive beats. Although the interval is measured in fractions of seconds, you can actually have a feel of the difference.

To have a sense of your HRV, place two fingers on your carotid artery (at the side of your neck) or on your wrist to find your pulse, and once you do, take deep breaths in and out. You will notice that the interval between your beats becomes longer (heart rate reduces) when you exhale while it becomes shorter (heart rate increases) when you inhale. Be aware that HRV can be influenced when exercising, which would create a much more consistent time lapse between beats. However, if at rest and you experience a high time variation between your breathing in and out, then it means you have a high HRV – a good sign of being able to cope with stress and a sign of having a good vagal tone (high vagal tone).

On the other hand, if at rest and you experience a low time variation between your breathing in and out, it means that you have a low HRV, mostly a fight or flight response to stress, which implies a low vagal tone – leading to your inability to cope with stress. If this state of low vagal tone persists for long, you will stand the risk of poor performance and health.

Although measuring your HRV using your pulse gives you a feel of what your HRV may be, it, however, does not provide you with an accurate HRV reading since it's difficult to detect actual variations in heartbeats without special technology. How you calculate your HRV is dependent on the technology, you wish to use.

One such common technology used today is the electrocardiogram (ECG) device. This device functions by picking up the electrical pulse from your heart's contraction. With the data retrieved, your HRV can be determined. Measuring your HRV using the ECG technology usually required you to visit a laboratory where complex machines and electrodes are placed over your body. But with technological advancement, this can simply be done at the comfort of your home using heart rate monitors such as the Polar H7 heart rate strap.

Also, a wearable smartwatch with an inbuilt ECG device has been validated in research as being a reliable method to measure your HRV. One such is the Apple Watch, which has been approved by the FDA. This even makes it very easy for lovers of Apple Watch to easily determine their HRV even on the go.

Another technology that doesn't use ECG to measure your HRV but instead requires an optical sensor to measure heartbeat intervals is the Photoplethysmography (PPG). PPG uses a light source and a photodetector at the surface of the skin to measure changes in blood volume. The well-known Oura ring uses PPG technology to determine the HRV.

The beauty of using either of these devices is that they are non-invasive which can be worn on your wrist, finger, or strapped around your chest to take measurement of your HRV even while asleep – this is very recommended because the longer the measurement while at rest with no distractions, the more reliable the data would be.

Interpreting Your Heart Rate Variability Result

There is no standard procedure for optimal HRV values, which is quite relatable given there are different methods to track and calculate it.

However, according to a 2016 study published in Health and Quality of Life Outcomes, low HRV are values that are <780ms while High HRV, as published in Sports Medicine Research, are values that are >=780 ms. HRV tends to be on the high side when a person is healthy and fit and how high this can be depend on the individual in question.

Because a number of factors such as age, gender, body functions, a person's lifestyle, and even hormones can affect the HRV reading, it is advisable that you do not compare your HRV value with that of others (even of the same gender). What you should rather do is focus on your own HRV and its trends. In addition, when using trends to compare your daily HRV values, measurement should be done using the same technology, and under similar conditions – preferably when sleeping at night since your body would be at rest.

Summing up, if the intervals of your heartbeat are constantly low, then you have a low HRV, and you would have a high HRV if the intervals are constantly high.

Increasing Your Vagal Tone

When your vagal tone is increased, it activates your parasympathetic nervous system, which for instance, would help your body relax faster after stress, your mood becomes more regulated, and your anxiety is better managed.

To a certain degree, the strength of your vagal tone is genetic, just like the mother who, during pregnancy, transferred her low vagal tone to her unborn child. This, however, does not imply that a low vagal tone cannot be changed and increased. Vagal tone can be increased using a number of methods such as undergoing some recommended natural exercises and practices e.g., deep breathing as well as the use of electrical stimulation methods, among others. Toward the tail end of this book, I would go deeper on these exercises and methods which you can use to increase your vagal tone.

A Short message from the Author:

Hey, I hope you are enjoying the book? I would love to hear your thoughts!

Many readers do not know how hard reviews are to come by and how much they help an author.

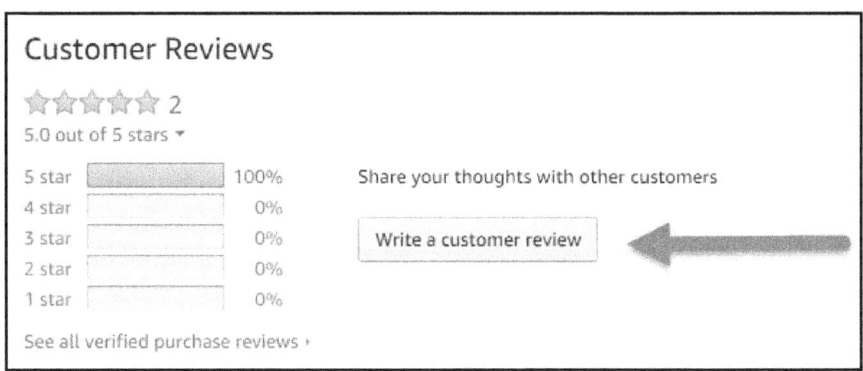

I would be incredibly grateful if you could take just 60 seconds to write a short review on Amazon, even if it is a few sentences!

>> Type this link https://amzn.to/2TiHu8O into your web browser to leave a quick review

Thanks for the time taken to share your thoughts!

Your review will genuinely make a difference for me and help gain exposure for my work.

Chapter 3

Conditions Associated with The Vagus Nerve

You probably are trying to understand why the dysfunction of the vagus nerve results in numerous diseases and health problems in the human body. Well, if you have assiduously followed my discussions from the beginning, you should already have your answer. The vagus nerve, as we already know, is the most complex cranial nerve, but not only that, it is also the largest network distribution of motor and sensory fibers within the human body compared to any of the 12 cranial nerves. It is as a result of this that the vagus nerve impacts a wide range of bodily functions such as gut-brain axis communication, neurotransmitter management, hormonal balance, and inflammation prevention, among many others. Therefore, any dysfunctions in the vagus nerve can have enormous effects throughout the body resulting in some of the many known diseases and health problems. That being said, it is important you know that most of these conditions outlined herein do not exist in isolation – meaning that if any of these conditions are taking place in the human body, it can also lead to further illness. For instance, obesity and inflammation are linked with cancers and diabetes just as anxiety or mood disorders could also result in depression.

Moving forward, let's take a look at some of the medical conditions that are associated with the vagus nerve.

Chronic Stress and Anxiety

When we subject ourselves to stressful situations such as the daily hassles of sitting in traffic for long hours, a pile of financial debt that keeps growing, stress arising from troubled relationships, unhappiness about your job, or even the stress to our body from the unhealthy foods we eat, the sympathetic nervous system becomes activated. If we are unable to turn off what activates the stress, not much time will pass by before these stress as little as it may seem compounds to become chronic stress, leading to health problems within our body. When we are stressed, two pathways become activated by the brain; the hypothalamus-pituitary-adrenal axis, and the brain-intestine axis.

During the fight or flight response, our brain would respond to stress and anxiety by increasing the production of Corticotropin-releasing hormone (CRF), the hormone involved in stress response. This hormone then travels from the hypothalamus to the pituitary gland, where they stimulate the release of adrenocorticotropic hormone (ACTH). This, in turn, then travels down the bloodstream to the adrenal glands to trigger cortisol and adrenaline induction – suppressors to our body's immune system and precursors of inflammation. This explains the reason why we easily fall ill when we are stressed and anxious, and eventually fall into depression, a mental disorder linked to inflammatory brain response. When cortisol is produced in a large amount, it causes the volume of the hippocampus to be reduced – this is the part of our brain that helps in the creation of new memories. Chronic stress and anxiety also lead to increased production of glutamate in the brain – a neurotransmitter that causes migraine, and also depression when it is produced in excess amount.

It is the inability of the vagus nerve to activate the parasympathetic rest and digest response when stressed or anxious that keeps the sympathetic nervous system up and running, thus making us respond with impulse and end up suffering from the effect.

Trauma, PTSD, and Depression

Witnessing a traumatic event such as natural disasters, an act of violence, abuse, or even a severe accident can affect one's mental wellbeing, which can lead to mental disorders. Whether we are directly involved in such incidents, or we have family or friends that were affected (killed or injured), or even learning of the incident through the media, we will still experience some level of emotional response. Irrespective of the nature of the trauma, it can have a long-lasting psychological effect on an individual.

The feelings we experience from traumatic events (such as sadness, mood swings, crying, social withdrawal, etc.) are part of the normal grieving and recovery process from any trauma. However, if these feelings remain unchecked and continue quite too often for an extended period of time and it starts to affect your daily living, you begin to abuse alcohol or illegal drugs, or you even have the thoughts of suicide, then they are symptoms of a more severe episode of depression. Also, some people respond to their trauma by exhibiting post-traumatic stress disorder (PTSD) tendencies. When this occurs, they find themselves reliving repeated flashbacks of the traumatic event, continuous nightmares, inability to focus, and largely they remain miserable. Depression and PTSD are signs of an out of control trauma – they are all closely related to each other.

The vagus nerve is actively involved in your emotional wellbeing, and it determines how much you will be emotionally affected by a traumatic event long after it is has ended.

A reduced heart rate variability (HRV) is a potential pointer of an increased emotional sensitivity following a trauma, an indication of an altered vagus nerve function, and impaired emotion regulation ability. Through the vagus nerve, the HRV parasympathetic regulation of the heart rate is measured. During safe non-traumatic situations, the vagus nerve reduces your heart rate. However, when responding to threats, the inhibiting heart-rate effect of the vagus nerve stops, which then allows the sympathetic nervous system to activate defense responses and increasing your heart rate. Continuous exposure to threats could affect the functioning of the vagus nerve over time –resulting in a reduced capability of your body to adjust to traumatic events. High HRV is a marker that your body has an increased emotion regulation ability even after experiencing a traumatic or stressful event, while low HRV clearly indicates the opposite. Low HRV has been linked to increased exposure to trauma, PTSD, depression, and delayed recovery from a stressful situation.

Lack of Social Interaction

Maintaining face to face social interaction engages your vagus nerve and increases your parasympathetic response, which is very important for your health. Imagine being isolated from people or being indoor for a whole week or more without having to have a face to face interaction with the outside world, your family members, partners, or even your close friends; you would most certainly become somewhat low spirited and moody. This is not a random feeling – your vagus nerve activates when you interact with people face to face and deactivates when you are isolated. Social connectedness improves heart rate variability (HRV), an indication of a high vagal tone.

A study published in Health Psychology in 2009 showed that participants who exhibited signs of depression and were isolated from social interactions had a low HRV. However, when they were engaged in face to face interactions with their partners, friends, or family members, their vagal parasympathetic response and HRV increased. This goes to demonstrate that having a face to face social interaction would improve the functioning of your vagus nerve while a lack of social interaction points to an underperforming vagus nerve.

Sleep Disorders and Disruptive Circadian Rhythm

A very common problem I have observed among people is an alteration of their body's natural sleep signaling or their circadian rhythm. The reason for this is partly because most people do not engage in more bodily activity during the day. A common routine during the day, for instance, would be to take the subway or drive our car to work, sit on our work desk for an extended number of hours, and at the close of work, we take the subway or drive our car back home.

Hardly do we see the sun during our time of work, and when we get back to our homes, we sit right in front of blue lights at night e.g., our mobile phones, computers or even our television – these blue lights falsely telling our brains that it is daytime. These blue light that is emitted from the screen of our electronic devices mimics the sun, tells our bodies it is time to get up, and instructs the pineal glands in our brains not to release melatonin (hormone promoting sleep).

Signals are transmitted by the vagus nerve from our circadian control center, which is high up in our brain. Disrupting the circadian flow affects the brain, and alterations in melatonin and any other hormone levels right before bedtime can result in problems with the vagus nerve.

Chronic Inflammation

If you have been following this book from the get-go, then you should know that I made it clear that a certain amount of inflammation after an injury or infection is not out of place, especially if it occurs temporarily. The sympathetic nervous system swiftly dives into action by triggering your body's immune system to respond immediately.

Inflammation is simply indicating your body's immune system is prepared to protect you from further harm so that you can heal. When inflammation occurs, blood vessels around the location of the injury or infection expands, releasing more immune system cells into the tissue surrounding the affected area. Temporal redness, swelling, and pain accompany the inflammation process – at this point, you have nothing to really worry about, so just relax, you are experiencing what is called acute inflammation.

Immediately your immune system reacts to the injury or infection by protecting it from further harm, the process of healing becomes activated by your parasympathetic nervous system in other for your body to relax and restore balance. Stress caused by the injury or infection becomes reduced, your heart and breathing rates revert to the status quo, and the inflammation starts to dissipate. However, if the parasympathetic nervous system is not functioning properly, your heart and breathing rates could remain high, and the inflammation can stay back to become chronic, paving the way to severe health problems such as rheumatoid arthritis or lupus among others – now this is where you should be worried, and very concerned, and obviously, our aim is to ensure it does not get to this point.

You must now, by now, that the vagus nerve is directly tied to your parasympathetic nervous system because of the important role it plays in stress reduction, lowering of high heart and breathing rates, and preventing any acute inflammation from being chronic. It also resets your immune system, preventing it from overreacting and over-responding, especially when there is no need to. If the vagus nerve is not in a healthy state, it can't counterbalance your sympathetic nervous system nor reset your immune system, which can result in a list of health conditions affiliated with chronic inflammation. Hence, keeping your vagus nerve in good and healthy condition is vital to your overall health and wellbeing, which can help protect you from the health problems that come with chronic inflammation.

Dysfunctional Breathing

Most of us unknowingly take our breathing for granted due to "how we breathe" as opposed to "how we should breathe."

What if I told you that you have dysfunctional breathing?

One of the most common reasons for vagus nerve missignaling is dysfunctional breathing.

When we were babies, we learned how to breathe automatically through the proper way i.e., using the diaphragm to breathe – this is known as belly breathing or abdominal breathing, a process of using the primary muscles (such as diaphragm muscle) to breathe normally instead of the secondary muscles (used for heavy breathing). As we inhale, our diaphragm contracts, pulls down, and decreases the pressure in our chest, and as we exhale, it relaxes and causes us to breathe out with our belly expanding in the process. This process of breathing helps our lungs to inflate very efficiently, allows the exchange of important oxygen and nutrients, as well as the removal of waste products. Interestingly when you breathe using your diaphragm, you are inadvertently activating your parasympathetic nervous system, through the signals of your vagus nerve, allowing your body to slow down, and heal during tense situations which are accompanied by reduced heart rate and blood pressure, relaxed muscles, improved digestion, decreased stress, increased energy levels, and mood elevation among others.

However, as we get older, our breathing becomes shallower (chest breathing) when we begin to use our secondary muscles (such as neck muscles, muscles between our ribs, and our chest muscles), which can cause pains in our neck, shoulder and severe headaches from overactive muscles. This process of breathing does not allow your lungs to inflate nor deflate properly, prevents the circulation of important nutrients and oxygen, as well as causing retention of more waste products in your body. Breathing with your chest for a long while could decrease how well your body responds to infection and disease, exerts more pressure on your heart, and makes fighting respiratory conditions more difficult. Chest breathing in contrast to diaphragm breathing activates your sympathetic nervous system, which raises your heart rate and blood pressure, increases the tension in your muscles, increases stress, and decreases your energy and mental clarity. When your body is subjected to stress for a long period of time, your immune system risks being inefficient, and as time passes by, the build-up of minor irritations can result in issues like anxiety, depression, and constant illness and infections.

Breathing properly is one of the simplest things to do for your health, but yet seen as very challenging by many. In subsequent sections where I focused on how to strengthen your vagal tone, I would describe how you can learn to breathe properly for a better and healthy living.

Dysfunctional Digestive System

Right off the bat, when the vagus nerve is dysfunctional, your digestion system stands the risk of being dysfunctional. Some of the signs of a dysfunctional digestion system may include heartburn or gastroesophageal reflux disease (GERD), and inflammatory bowel disease (IBD) such as ulcerative colitis which can prevent your body from healing small intestine bacterial overgrowth (SIBO), a common cause of irritable bowel syndrome (IBS).

The vagus nerve tells your stomach to release digestive acids and enzymes and to begin the gut movement. When you chew your food, you begin the process of mixing the fibers in your food with the digestive acids and enzymes which start to breakdown the food before it gets to your stomach and before traveling down to your small and large intestines.

When the vagus nerve is not receiving or transmitting the right signals, the flow of food mixed with digestive acid and enzymes via the gut is slowed. The implication of this is that bacteria overgrowths, yeast or parasite, including used up hormones and toxins your body worked to remove from your body system, are traveling through your gut at a slow rate. Your body's exposure to these bacteria increases the risk of having IBS and SIBO, which can potentially worsen any infections already present in your body.

Dysfunctional Heart Rate

The number of times the heart beats per minute is referred to as the heart rate, and it is directly associated with the workload the heart is subjected to as we go about our daily life activities.

When the body is at rest (i.e., relaxed for a given amount of time), the resting heart rate can be measured. The normal resting heart rate for most people falls within the range of 60-100 beats per minute (bpm). However, for athletics, it is normal if it falls within 40-60 bpm. Dysfunctional heart rate or abnormal heart rhythms describes a heart that is beating too fast (above 100 bpm) or too slow (below 60 bpm).

The electrical signals of the sympathetic nervous system control the heart rate and release the hormones (epinephrine and norepinephrine) to increase the heart rate, while the parasympathetic nervous system causes the release of acetylcholine hormone through the vagus nerve to reduce the heart rate. In other words, the strength of your vagus nerve is determined by how low your resting heart rate is. Factors such as stress, excitement, or even exercising may elevate your heart rate temporarily while engaging in deep breaths, or meditation, for instance, can help slow your heart rate. When your heartbeat is unable to revert to its normal resting heart rate after a stressful event or activity, then this may be a pointer of a dysfunctional vagus nerve. When you are able to calm your nerves and slow down your heart after stress, then it is a marker you have a strong vagus nerve. The opposite is someone with a dysfunctional vagus nerve. An abnormally low heart rate (called bradycardia) can also occur if the vagus nerve is overactive. Bradycardia is when the resting heart rate is below 60 beats per minute, which is healthy and normal, especially for athletics, whose resting heart rate ranges from 40-60, as earlier mentioned. However, problems can be caused by bradycardia if the heart rate is so low that the heart cannot pump enough blood to supply the needs of the body. How well you are able to handle stressful situations would determine how well your vagus nerve would respond. If you are unable to function in a stressful situation, then an overactive vagus nerve can also occur. This makes sense especially if stress is over-activated causing your body to over-activate your vagus nerve i.e., a lot of chemicals slowing your heart rate and lowering your blood pressure, which means less blood circulation to the brain, making you lose consciousness momentarily, and causing you to faint – a term known as vasovagal syncope. Although vasovagal syncope is a sign of improper balance within the autonomic nervous system (i.e., between the sympathetic and parasympathetic nervous system), the imbalance is, however, not the single cause. Different causes exist and vary between young and old individuals. Vasovagal syncope is not life-threatening except someone faints quite too often, and if that is the case, it is often a sign of an immune issue that is yet to be diagnosed. Conducting a functional lab test and neurology can shed more light on the potential root cause, which is, in most cases, a symptom that the nerves in the autonomic nervous system and overactivation of the vagus nerve are not functioning properly.

Chapter 4

Substances That May Affect Your Vagus Nerve

While it is important for you to recognize certain factors that could interfere with the healthy functioning of your vagus nerve such as stress, anxiety, smoking, alcoholism, and poor sleeping habits among others, you should also keep watch of certain chemical substances that enters your body aside from the food you eat. You will be shocked that some of the substances you presumed to be unharmful can potentially cause severe damage to your vagus nerve.

Let's have a look at some of these substances.

Botox

It is a known fact that Botox (botulinum toxin) has several vital medical applications, and prominent amongst them is its usage in reducing lines and facial wrinkles by paralyzing the underlying muscles. Although Botox is applied in the treatment of some medical conditions, you should also be aware that it is a powerful and dangerous toxin which, when used inappropriately, can result in Botulism, an illness that causes respiratory failure, and eventually lead to death. A study shows that a gram of botulinum toxin has the capacity to kill over a million people, and two kilograms could potentially exterminate the entire human population – this is how dangerous it is.

So then, how can Botox cause damage to your vagus nerve?

When Botox is injected into the body, one of its targets is to stop the production of the chemical neurotransmitter called acetylcholine. Acetylcholine production is stimulated by the vagus nerve, which, when released, causes our muscles to contract, regulates our endocrine system, and aids in learning and memory formation, among others. When the vagus nerve does not stimulate the release of acetylcholine, our nerves will fail to receive signals, which would result in some problems such as myasthenia gravis, a disorder that affects the voluntary muscle contraction of the face, neck, mouth, and eyes. Sufferers of this disorder would have difficulty breathing, swallowing, and speaking. Other problems that may arise are double vision, and droopy eyelids.

As you can see, Botox has far too severe consequences when used wrongly. Can you imagine not being able to breathe or swallow? This can either lead to death or problems with some of your vital organs.

In using Botox, you should be well educated on the risks it has to your health. Should you decided to further its usage in treating any medical condition, ensure to choose an experienced and certified doctor to perform the Botox procedure, and also adhere to the doctor's instructions after the surgery.

Certain Antibiotics

There appears to be a thin line between certain antibiotics, most especially fluoroquinolone and its effect on the vagus nerve. Unfortunately, not enough research has been conducted and released on how fluoroquinolones can impact the vagus nerve.

However, I would provide you with my perspective on this.

Fluoroquinolones (ciprofloxacin, levofloxacin, moxifloxacin, and its other brands) are antibiotics used commonly in the treatment of several bacteria-related illnesses, most especially, respiratory and urinary tract infections. The FDA in 2013 strengthened its warning that fluoroquinolones could cause severe and permanent nerve damage called peripheral neuropathy and required updates to drug labels to reflect this risk.

Peripheral neuropathy arises when nerves are damaged and unable to send signals from the brain and spinal cord to the muscles and other parts of the body. It would interest you to know that the autonomic nervous system, risk being damaged by fluoroquinolone antibiotics.

Having established that peripheral neuropathy causes damage to the nerves, and given our knowledge that the vagus nerve is the longest of all 12 nerves that connect to multiple organs in our body from the brain and that this same nerve is part of the autonomic nervous system, there is no doubt that fluoroquinolones can cause damage to the vagus nerve. You might disapprove of my conclusion from this theory due to lack of adequate facts and data, but personally, I know this because once when I had a severe reaction to ciprofloxacin, each of those body functions controlled by the vagus nerve was affected.

Though no scientific evidence is yet to be published in support of this theory, my interactions with several patients that experienced similar symptoms prove this theory is valid. It took the FDA about 30 years to recognize the effect of fluoroquinolones, so I would not be swift to disregard its possible effect on the autonomic nervous system and, by extension, its effect on the vagus nerve. I suspect the reason the FDA has not investigated the autonomic neuropathy's possible association with fluoroquinolones is because the problems that arise from the autonomic nervous system are difficult to describe and detect, but most importantly, it hasn't gotten to the top list of complaints in the AERS database (where FDA receives medication error complaints and reports).

Research also shows that administering fluoroquinolones to patients with a history of myasthenia gravis (earlier discussed) can exacerbate this disorder, and can lead to death. Hence, administering fluoroquinolone antibiotics to such patients should be avoided.

This by no means implies that fluoroquinolone antibiotics should not be administered when the need arises, but it should be used in addition to probiotics, which is used to add vital bacteria into the body, which the fluoroquinolone antibiotics may have removed. Nonetheless, always consult with your doctor and be well educated on the risks of using fluoroquinolones.

Heavy Metals

Heavy metals such as arsenic, cadmium, copper, iron, lead, mercury, and zinc, among others, are all around us. They can be found in the food we eat, the water we drink, the ground we walk on, the injections we receive into our body, and in our everyday cosmetic care products, to say the least. Not all of these metals are toxic to our bodies. For instance, our bodies require a small amount of copper, zinc, and iron to perform some physiological and biological activities in order to keep us healthy. High amounts of heavy metals, in general, can have a severe impact on our health, which can damage and disrupt the functioning of our internal organs such as the kidney, lungs, and liver, to mention but a few. Of all the heavy metals, mercury poses the most threat to our body.

How then does mercury affect the vagus nerve?

Just like Botox, which inhibits the production of acetylcholine, research also validates the same for mercury. Mercury prevents the action of acetylcholine. For instance, when mercury finds its way to the heart muscle receptors, the heart muscle would be unable to receive the vagus nerve electrical signal needed for contraction. The implication of this could result in cardiovascular problems such as cardiac arrest.

It is important to get in touch with your doctor to test for the amount of mercury in your body. If your body has a high amount of mercury, request to undergo a mercury detox. Although trace amounts of mercury can be found in the food we eat, which our body can control, you should take additional steps to minimize your exposure to high mercury. Some of which are but not limited to the following:

- Avoiding fishes with high mercury such as tuna and swordfish
- Avoiding amalgam fillings
- Avoiding skin-lightening products and other cosmetics with high mercury concentration
- Using water filters that are designed to filter mercury

- Wearing gloves when digging the soil of your gardens to limit the absorption of mercury into your skin

Excess Sugar Intake

Some foods, like sugar, can also cause inflammation in the body, which is normal. However, taking excess added sugar poses severe health risks, such as high blood pressure and diabetes – a disease characterized by an increased blood sugar level, which potentially leads to the damage of the blood vessels, heart, kidneys, and nerves. Unfortunately, high blood pressure and diabetes are not the only concern that poses a risk to the human body; chronic inflammation can also result from the intake of excess added sugar. Don't get me wrong, inflammation is a normal part of our body's healing process in which some sugar-laden foods could cause, which is very normal. However, consuming excess sugar (added sugar and not natural sugar) that goes unchecked could result in chronic inflammation, which is the root cause of many chronic diseases. These inflammations can likewise disrupt the body's nervous systems from signaling information across different parts of the body.

Preventing interruptions to our body's communication system is thus vital to the healthy functioning of the body, which is why you should be careful enough to watch the amount of added sugar you allow into your body.

Being watchful of the substances mentioned herein and adhering to the do's and don'ts are a vital part of ensuring your vagus nerve is not damaged but alive and kicking. That being said, you could potentially slip and fall victim to these substances, which could cause severe damage to your vagus nerve. It is important to note that these substances are only a few of what could cause damage to your vagus nerve. Other factors, as discussed throughout this book, can also contribute to the malfunctioning of your vagus nerve. This is the more reason why you need to be well informed on how to stimulate the vagus nerve to fight against the health problems that may arise from either these substances or the other factors already discussed.

How you can stimulate this nerve is our focus for the next chapter.

The end… almost!

Hey! We've made it to the final chapter of this book, and I hope you've enjoyed it so far.

If you have not done so yet, I would be incredibly thankful if you could take just a minute to leave a quick review on Amazon

Reviews are not easy to come by, and as an independent author with a little marketing budget, I rely on you, my readers, to leave a short review on Amazon.

Even if it is just a sentence or two!

Customer Reviews

★★★★★ 2
5.0 out of 5 stars ▼

5 star	▬▬▬▬	100%
4 star		0%
3 star		0%
2 star		0%
1 star		0%

See all verified purchase reviews ›

Share your thoughts with other customers

[Write a customer review] ⬅

So if you really enjoyed this book, please...

>> Type this link https://amzn.to/2TiHu8O into your web browser to leave a brief review on Amazon.

I truly appreciate your effort to leave your review, as it truly makes a huge difference.

Thanks once again from the depth of my heart for purchasing this book and reading it to the end

Chapter 5

Stimulating Your Vagus Nerve

When you develop a deep understanding of how your vagus nerve works, you will find it possible to work with your nervous system instead of feeling trapped when it works against you. It wouldn't be out of place to mention that I have enjoyed a sound physical and mental health over the years (which I still do), simply because I understood the incredible effect stimulating my vagus nerve had on my overall wellbeing.

Throughout the course of this book, I shed several lights on the anatomy of the vagus nerve, its importance to your physical and mental wellbeing, the causes of an impaired vagus nerve, the health conditions associated with it, and why it is important to increase the tone and strength of your vagus nerve. In this chapter, I would reveal in detail what you should do to increase the tone of your vagus nerve vis-a-vis engaging in specific natural exercises and practices, passive methods of stimulation, as well as recommended food and dietary supplements. Be aware that some of these methods may seem offbeat, but what I am about to reveal are based on science and are all found to be very effective at increasing your vagal tone.

Without further ado, let's dive in.

Natural Exercises and Practices

Deep and Slow Breathing

Earlier, I discussed the effect of dysfunctional breathing mostly because we breathe through our chest instead of our diaphragm. In this section, I would be describing how you can start breathing the proper way using the deep and slow diaphragmatic breathing technique.

But before then...

Many of us don't breathe properly while at rest, we breathe at a very fast pace (about 10-14 breaths per minute instead of taking about 5-7 breaths per minute). When this happens, we short change ourselves from the power the vagus nerve has on our wellbeing. When you take a deep, slow breath, your vagus nerve becomes stimulated by lowering your sympathetic (fight or flight) nervous system and activating your parasympathetic (rest and digest) nervous system. When this happens, your heart rate, blood pressure, and any feelings of anxiety become reduced.

Deep and slow breathing exercises can also help divert your attention away from the sensation of pain.

How do I mean?

If you focus your attention on the rhythm of your breathing, you won't feel the sensation of your pain since you are not focused on the pain itself. On the flip side, when you focus on the pain, you will be forced to hold our breath. Anytime you hold your breath, the fight or flight response gets activated, which then increases not just the sensation of pain but also sensations of stiffness, fear, and anxiety. To practice deep and slow breathing, you must learn to breathe through your diaphragm and not through your chest – this drains your energy and makes you anxious, among others.

To start breathing from your diaphragm, proceed as follows:

- Get comfortable by either sitting on a chair while resting your head, neck, and shoulders against the back of the chair or laying your back against the floor or bed, supported by a pillow to your head and feet.
- Lay one of your hand on your upper chest and the other on your belly.

- Shut your eyes and breathe in deeply and slowly into your belly via your nose (i.e., to expand your diaphragm) to the count of five, take a pause then

- Slowly exhale through your mouth to the count of ten

- Repeat the same process for about 5-10 minutes

Ideally, your breath has to be reduced to 5-7 breaths per minute to activate the parasympathetic rest and digest mode. As your breath per minute is reduced and the parasympathetic mode gets activated, your muscles become relaxed, causing all sensations of pain, fear, anxiety, or even worries to be lowered. When this happens, the supply of oxygen to the cells of your body increases which then help to produce your body's feel–good hormones called endorphins.

You can enhance your breathing experience as you inhale while imagining the beauty of being loved or the air being filled with peace and calm, and as you exhale, imagine reciprocating that same love or the air leaving with any sensations of pain, or anxiety. There is nothing really mysterious about this breathing technique. This is an ancient technique that has been practiced for decades by the Tibetan monks, which can also help improve your memory, tackle depression, as well as boost your immune system – at a price of zero dollars.

How often you decide to practice this breathing technique solely depends on you. You can either make it a daily routine or anytime you feel on edge. However, I recommend the former so that you not only train yourself to stop breathing through your chest but also be able to easily adapt to the breathing technique, making it more easy to initiate whenever you are on edge. Practicing deep, slow, and diaphragmatic breathing to activate your vagus nerve can perform wonders for your physical and mental wellbeing.

Humming or Chanting

The vagus nerve fibers originating from the brainstem connects your larynx (voice box) and the muscles behind your throat, and it is responsible for governing the movement of your vocal cords. As a matter of fact, impairment of the vagus nerve is what causes vocal paralysis. Humming or chanting have been proven to stimulate the vagus nerve, and awakening the laryngeal muscles, thereby increasing the vagal tone. A study performed by Dr. Stephen Porges showed that the vibrations produced from humming or chanting aloud wake up your vagus nerve so that it comes online. To begin stimulating your vagus nerve through this practice, all you need to do is chant the word "OM," "home," "hum," or "hmmm," while stretching the "mmm" sound for as long as possible (say 10 secs or more). You can observe and enjoy the vibration sensations produced in your head, chest, throat, ear, and even throughout your body. Continue humming or chanting for about 10-15 minutes per session, with up to 2 sessions in a day or as many as you can perform per day.

This exercise is most productive when performed on a daily basis. Humming or chanting affords us the ability to regulate our breath and calm down our thoughts, especially during or after a stressful event. It is also shown to improve the level of digestion and inflammation in the body.

Singing

Just like humming or chanting, singing also activates the vagus nerve and awakens the laryngeal muscles. Singing is like activating a vagal pump to send out waves of relaxation. I usually sing my favorite songs at the top of my voice anytime I feel moody, and a surge of positive energy immediately flows through my body, calming my frayed nerves. It does not matter whether you choose to sing alone or in unison (in a church or with a group of friends), either of such would activate the vagus nerve function, increase relaxation and elevate your mood, and also increase your heart rate variability (HRV).

Humor Therapy

Laughing is one very easy way to stimulate the vagus nerve. It is a natural immune booster to the body, which, by research, is also found to increase one's heart rate variability (HRV). Laughing increases the movement of your diaphragm and the pressure on your abdomen (stomach). Because the vagus nerve travels from the brainstem, passing through the diaphragm, these movements would activate your rest and digest the parasympathetic nervous system that sends signals to your body to relax. When you laugh, you are typically activating your rest and digest the nervous system to lower your stress hormones and trigger the release of the body's painkillers, such as endorphins (a feel-good hormone). Stepping out for a comedy show, watching a comedy film, or simply joking around with families and friends is one sure way to get started. However, you don't necessarily need to laugh aloud to have a feel of the soothing relief laughter can bring when your vagus nerve is stimulated. You can also find something in your office that can make you smile, watch a humorous television program, read humorous books or anything that makes you chuckle on the inside – all are just as therapeutic as laughing out loud.

Gargling

The gargling technique was popularized by Dr. Datis Kharrazian, which simply means holding and pouring a liquid (i.e., water) into the mouth, and to the back of the throat while moving it around aggressively to make a gurgling sound.

When you gargle, the pharyngeal muscles (muscles at the back of your throat) contracts, causing the activation of your vagus nerve – it is often described as "sprints" for your vagus nerve. For gargling to be effective, you would need to gargle aggressively and loudly, to the point where tears come into your eyes, and if it doesn't, keep going at it until you do. This actually shows that you have activated your vagus nerve. This can be pretty difficult to do at first, especially if your vagal tone is weak. Ideally, you should be gargling for up to 5 minutes, three times per day. However, start with a shorter time and build up gradually. Adding salt to the water when you are about to gargle has been shown to produce an anti-bacteria impact that can help eliminate unwanted bacteria from the mouth and respiratory tract.

Gargling on a daily basis would help increase your vagus nerve responsiveness to regulate relaxation, metabolism, and digestion, and it has also been demonstrated to improve memory performance.

Gag Reflex

Gag reflex, just like gargling, is another way to stimulate the pharyngeal muscles that the vagus nerve innervates, and is often described as "push-ups" for your vagus nerve. Gag reflex (also called pharyngeal reflex) occurs when the back of your tongue or even the roof of your mouth is touched by an object that causes the back of your throat to contract. Gag reflex helps protect us from choking as well as helping to govern the transition of food from liquid to solid during infancy. You can use a tongue depressor, your toothbrush, or any convenient but safe object to activate the gag reflex. Ideally, for this exercise to produce the much-needed change such as increasing your vagal tone, it should be done several times (i.e., 5-10) on a daily basis, spanning several weeks and mostly importantly it should be done until tear comes into your eyes (a sign that your vagus nerve has been stimulated). As a precautionary measure, gently press whatever object you choose to use on the back of your tongue, then push down gradually to the back of your throat to activate the gag reflex. This is to prevent you from poking the back of your throat with the object and hurting yourself. Activating the gag reflex immediately fires up the vagus nerve to keep sending signals that the body requires.

Exposure to Cold

Cold exposure has been described to activate the vagus nerve. Studies show that when you regularly expose your body to cold, your body adjusts to the cold, causing a decrease in the activity of the fight or flight nervous system while increasing the rest and digest nervous system activity.

Immersion of the face in cold water proves to be a simple but yet effective way to activate the parasympathetic nervous system after a stressful activity such as an exercise or when you generally feel worn out. For the cold water face immersion to be very effective, it is recommended that you remain seated, bending your head forward into a cold water basin at a temperature of about 10-12°C. Your face should be immersed such that your forehead, your eyes, and two-thirds of your cheeks are also submerged in the water.

Coldwater showers can also be taken, likewise finishing your warm water shower with at 30 seconds or more of cold water. Alternatively, you can put some cubes of ice in a sealed bag, and then hold it up against your face, while holding your breath for some time, or you can take a swim in a cold water pool - these are all great ways to get your vagus nerve online.

I have experimented with all these techniques, and I have found them to be quite exhilarating. Often times, I take cold showers and go outside, especially when the temperature is cold, with minimal clothing. If you reside in a cold winter climate area, then it would be great if you could take a walkout on a frigid day. Otherwise, try using cold therapy in a cryo-chamber (a tank of the size of a human, filled with nitrogen-cooled air) if you can afford it – the majority of athletes and performers such as Tony Robbins uses this method.

These methods, as described, can easily stimulate an unresponsive vagus nerve when done regularly, helping to reduce your heart rate, blood pressure, and lowering your stress hormone levels – overall boosting your immune system.

Sudarshan Kriya Yoga

As shown by research, yoga (a mind-body relaxation practice) can stimulate the vagus nerve by elevating your parasympathetic activity and reducing inappropriate activation of your autonomic activity. A clinical trial conducted on irritable bowel syndrome (IBS) patients showed that the overactivation of the sympathetic nervous system was the main contributing cause of the disease. Yoga, which increases the parasympathetic activity of the nervous system, proved to be a remedial therapy for IBS.

The sudarshan kriya, asana, pranayama, and nadi shodhana yoga has been found by scientists to be extremely effective at stimulating the vagus nerve. However, one popular yoga technique shown to be very effective and scientifically proven to stimulate the vagus nerve naturally is the sudarshan kriya Yoga, a type of mind-body relaxation breathing technique. This technique harmonizes the body, the mind, and emotions through specific breathing rhythms to diffuse stress, fatigue, as well as negative emotions such as anger, depression, and frustration. In a scientific study conducted, it was shown that a 68%–73% success rate was recorded in its treatment of depression, and also shown to help treat people with PTSD. Another study showed that practicing sudarshan kriya led to a significant drop in cortisol levels (stress hormone), suggesting that continuous practice of this yoga technique would result in a greater level of stress resistance and relaxation.

Generally, practicing sudarshan kriya yoga increases the GABA level (a calming neurotransmitter in the brain that inhibits stress, anxiety, and mood swings) by directly stimulating vagal afferent fibers, which in turn increases the parasympathetic nervous system activity—making it very helpful for people who struggle with anxiety, depression, and PTSD.

Loving Kindness Meditation

Loving-kindness meditation has been shown to be very effective in stimulating the vagus nerve and increasing heart rate variability. Loving-kindness meditation helps people look beyond themselves and become more aware of others by promoting a feeling of goodwill toward their needs, struggles, and desires.

To practice loving-kindness meditation, you are required to sit in silence for a given amount of time while cultivating feelings of warmth, tenderness, and compassion toward others by silently repeating phrases to yourself that is aimed at wishing them love, strength, and general wellbeing. A study conducted in 2010 by Barbara Fredrickson, a foremost researcher of positive emotions, showed that an increased positive emotion resulted in increased social closeness and a high vagal tone. And since social connection and bonds are mediated by vagal tone, those whose vagal tone increased were suddenly able to experience more moments of love toward others in subsequent times.

Regular practicing of loving-kindness meditation increases one's capacity to love even more, which can also translate into better health given that high vagal tone is associated with reduced risk of inflammation, cardiovascular disease, stroke, and even better mood among others.

Exposure to Sunlight

Sunlight exposure affects the cellular functioning of our body, which is genetically wired to function based on how much sunlight we are exposed to. When you spend your whole day away from the sun whether commuting to work via subways, or driving to work, or anywhere for that matter, and then returning home late in the evening from your busy work or activity without having enough skin to eye contact with the sun, you are more often depriving your cells from performing optimally.

Exposing your eye and skin to the sun is all about your circadian rhythm and having a good restful sleep at night. For instance, when light comes in contact with your eye (I don't mean looking directly into the sun), the melanopsin protein in the retina detects the light using vitamin A, and then it signals the brain that it is day time. But when it is nightfall, this signal is then turned off. Studies show that when you expose your eye and skin to sunlight, the melatonin (sleep hormone) levels increase at night.

Exposure to sunlight is linked to boosting serotonin production in the brain, and also facilitates your circadian rhythm and vagus nerve to regulate your heart rate. Hence, it is recommended that you go outside more often on a sunny day to feel the sun's warmth.

Precaution, however, should be taken when exposed to sunlight because having too much of the sun's rays (UVA and UVB) can be harmful to you. Instead, you should strike a balance between these rays. UVA and UVB rays are strongest between 10 a.m and 4 p.m, therefore the best times for sunlight exposure should be within 30 minutes of sunrise (2-3 times in the day) and 30 minutes of sunset.

Coffee Enema

A coffee enema is basically used for detoxification and gut motility, i.e., to cleanse your bowels and relieve constipation. When you take a coffee enema, the caffeine it contains will stimulate the release of the cholinergic receptor (in particular, the nicotinic receptor) in the gut, which then stimulates the movement and expansion of your bowel, thus activating your vagus nerve. This is particularly effective if high concentration of caffeine is taken, which then creates the urge to have a bowel movement. The key is to resist the urge and try holding it for as long as possible. By resisting the urge, you are actually training your brain and vagus nerve to learn how to activate your gut motility. If you do this regularly with a coffee enema, after a while, your vagus nerve would have learned how to release stools from your bowel without depending on coffee enema. At first, it may be difficult to keep up with, especially if your vagal tone is low, but with time, it becomes easier. If you suffer from chronic constipation and poor liver detoxification, there is no doubt that the process of taking coffee enema and resisting the urge would help detoxify your body and clear out your bowels very efficiently.

Personally, I used coffee enema on a daily basis for several months when I underwent an intensive program for detoxification while also resisting the urge. Over time, it helped me wean off any dependency on them, thus enabling my vagus nerve to activate my gut motility and restoring healthy bowel movements when I needed to detoxify and cleanse my bowels.

Overall, when it comes to your health, most especially the health of your gut, nothing is more critical than attending to your brain health and stimulating your vagal nerve response. By doing so, your gastrointestinal motility can be improved, thereby eliminating constipation and poor detoxification.

Massage

Having a massage is another way to stimulate your vagus nerve. I always visit the spa every weekend for some massage treatment, especially after a very stressful weekday just to destress my body, and the feeling afterward is always soothing and invigorating. Getting a massage instantly makes you relaxed, and when you are relaxed, your parasympathetic rest and digest response gets triggered. Anytime you activate your parasympathetic nervous system, you inadvertently stimulate your vagus nerve.

Massaging several areas of your body, most especially along your carotid artery (the side of your neck where a pulse is checked) or your foot is highly efficient for vagus nerve stimulation. A study shows that massage done to the throat region are found to reduce seizures while foot massages when performed can be helpful to increase your heart rate variability (HRV) and vagal activity, while also reducing your heart rate and blood pressure, all of which minimizes the risk of heart diseases. If you have never gone to the spa to get a massage, I strongly recommend that you do, but if you are not financially buoyant to visit the spa, you can do so at the comfort of your home. Your spouse, partner, or someone you are comfortable with can help massage your foot. However, doing a carotid artery massage at home by an unprofessional is not recommended because it could possibly lead to fainting.

Movement or Exercise

Most brain health professionals recommend movement or exercise as their top piece of advice for maximum brain health functioning. Exercise has been found to stimulate the vagus nerve which then helps increase the brain's growth hormone, supports the brain's energy as well as help reverse cognitive decline – which clearly points to the positive effects it has on our brain and overall mental health. Many of us do not put our bodies to work, with no actual movement or exercise to warm up our bodies. Most times, we are in a fixed spot, sitting for long periods at work, in the car, on the couch at home, or any other place for that matter without really moving or exercising our body for a good amount of time. Its high time you started a routine of movement or exercise that increases your heart rate and, by so doing, improves your parasympathetic rest and digest system, as well as training your body to easily recover from stress.

To get started, you can choose whatever movement or exercise that works best for you. Walking, weightlifting and sprinting are some of the best exercises you can start with. However, it is recommended that you choose an exercise or sporting activity that you love and enjoy to enable you to keep at it consistently.

Here is my exercise routine:

- Heavy weightlifting (4 times per week)
- High-intensity sprinting (2 times per week)
- Walking every day for 30-60 minutes

Food and Dietary Supplement

Probiotics

Earlier in this book, I discussed how the vagus nerve facilitates communication between our gut and the brain, and the role the microbiome (bacteria) in our gut plays with regard to our physical and mental health. The healthy bacteria present in our gut are what stimulates the positive feedback loop to our brain via the Vagus nerve. What I mean to say is that these bacteria in our gut basically stimulates the release of various neurotransmitters (such as Serotonin, Dopamine, and GABA, which are partly responsible for how we feel and what we think) to our brain, and mediated by the vagus nerve. Our body has lots of bacteria, both those that are good and those that are bad. Probiotics are live microorganisms (usually bacteria) that are found in food or supplements and are intended to reproduce, maintain and or improve the healthiness of the good bacteria in our body such as that found in our gut.

Lactobacillus Rhamnosus and Bifidobacterium Longum are the two main species that the majority of probiotic supplements are made of. For instance, research showed that probiotics stimulate the production of important neurotransmitters that impacts our mental health, and Lactobacillus Rhamnosus is one such probiotic, which was found to improve the Gamma-Aminobutyric Acid (GABA) neurotransmitter levels in the brain. It was found that the vagus nerve was stimulated by this probiotic bacteria, which in turn, stimulated the production of GABA. GABA has several functions it performs in the body, among which is to control anxiety and improve our mood. Bifidobacterium Longum also showed to normalize anxiety-like behavior in a clinical test conducted.

The vagus nerve essentially reads the gut microbiome, initiating a response to regulate inflammation based on whether it detects pathogenic or non-pathogenic bacteria. Probiotics help the vagus nerve to fight off inflammation, and when the gut microbiome is overrun by pathogenic (bad) bacteria, the result is the creation of the breeding ground for inflammation.

It is important you test your gut microbiome to know how healthy your gut is and also to determine if there are sufficient levels of probiotics in your gut. Probiotics in the gut microbiome can have a positive health impact on your immune system, and other factors that may reduce your vagal tone.

Fermented foods such as yogurt, kefir, sauerkraut, cheese, kimchi, sauerkraut, kombucha, and miso are known to be rich in probiotics. So, you may want to incorporate these foods as part of your diet. Nonetheless, always consult a health practitioner who is familiar with probiotics before you start or stop the intake of any probiotic-based supplement or food.

Omega-3 Fatty Acids

Omega-3 fatty acids are essential fats our body requires, which the body itself cannot produce, but rather, gotten from foods that are high in omega 3 such as salmon fish, walnuts, flaxseed, soybean oil, and seaweed. There is a lot of negativity pertaining to fatty foods. However, we all need healthy fat diets for our mental health, but the source of the fats we consume also matter. Research show that when you consume omega 3 fatty acids (which are primarily found in fish, most especially, fatty fish, e.g., salmon), it turns on your parasympathetic mode, thereby increasing your vagal tone and activity. To bring a balance to our system, we need about three times the amount of omega-3 fatty acids else, the vagal tone of our vagus nerve would decline.

While taking eicosapentaenoic acid (EPA), a type of omega-3 fatty acid important for cellular function, also ensure to get enough docosahexaenoic acid (DHA) in your diet. This is because DHA accounts for about 90% of the omega-3 fats in our brain. Nonetheless, our body can only produce a little amount of DHA from other fatty acids; hence, it has to be consumed from food or supplement. So, make sure you have a good amount of fish, oil, nuts, and or seeds that are high in omega 3 in other to get a high-quality DHA to stimulate your vagus nerve.

DHA and EPA are the two key types of omega- 3 fatty acids. Fish diets that are rich in DHA and EPA are salmon, mackerel, seabass, oysters, shrimp, and sardines, while seaweed and algae are vegetable diets that also contain DHA and EPA.

If you are unable to meet your omega-3 dietary requirements, then you can benefit from taking omega-3 supplements. There are many types of omega-3 supplements rich in DHA and EPA that you can choose from, such as fish oil, cod liver oil, krill oil, and algae oil. Personally, I eat a lot of salmon fish, supplemented with krill oil, in order to get my parasympathetic mode stimulated. Both DHA and EPA can help reduce inflammation as well as the risk of chronic diseases, such as heart disease.

Omega-3 fatty acid has been shown to help overcome addiction, reverse decline in cognitive ability, and even help to repair leaky brain. It has also been shown to increase heart rate variability in obese children, making it all too important for impacting several aspects of our mental health and overall wellness.

Passive Methods of Stimulation

Auricular Acupuncture

Really and truly, I am a very big fan of auricular (ear) acupuncture, a form of ancient alternative medicine that involves the insertion of needles into specific points on the ear. As earlier discussed, the vagus nerve is sensitive to touch felt on the skin of the ear, especially the external parts and receives sensory information via its auricular branch. Using the auricular acupuncture technique can, therefore, send sensory information to the vagus nerve via the auricular branch, which, in turn, causes a stimulation of the vagus nerve. This has also been validated by research and has been shown to increase vagal activity and tone, as well as help in the treatment of depression, anxiety, epilepsy, and digestive disorders.

There has been a growing trend in recent times, where the vagus nerve can be stimulated by a transcutaneous (non-invasive) electrical device applied to the external part of the ear, which was found to increase the parasympathetic rest and digest response and reduce the sympathetic fight or flight response. A reported study (Addorisio et al., 2019) showed that using a transcutaneous electrical device applied to certain parts of the ear to stimulate the vagus nerve activated the rest and digest nervous system in a way that drastically reduced inflammation.

Auricular acupuncture and the surgically implanted vagus nerve stimulation devices (to be discussed shortly) both provide the same effect. So, if you want to avoid surgical implants that are not invasive, then I would recommend you go with acupuncture, which is what I would personally go for at any time.

On a lighter note, it was once reported that a man passed on from a very low heart rate after vagus nerve stimulation using acupuncture. In light of this, I strongly advise that you work with a certified acupuncture practitioner and also notify your doctor if you intend to see an acupuncturist.

Chiropractor Care

The healthiness of the vagus nerve is very important to chiropractors because the vagus nerve is intimately associated with the spine and upper neck. The role the spinal health plays in coordinating the health of the vagus nerve is very significant. If the positioning of the spine and its ability to move freely becomes altered, the information that travels along the spinal nerves become interrupted. This is particularly noticed when you sit for long hours at work, busy working with your computer and hardly moving around. The result is a sensation of pain, mostly at your back and neck.

For better activity of the vagus nerve, chiropractors ensure the spines are well aligned and move freely. For instance, a study shows that the manipulation of the spine of a patient with pain (from lack of movement) at the back and neck by a chiropractor significantly improved the activity of the vagus nerve, resulting in reduced blood pressure and high heart rate variability (HRV). However, to experience sustained improvements in blood pressure and HRV, I strongly recommended that regular chiropractic care be administered. When in pain, chiropractic care can be a very effective method to increase your parasympathetic and vagus nerve activity.

Electrical Stimulation

Over the years, scientists have been exploring the influence of the nerve on the brain. One of the very complicated and interesting nerve they explored is the vagus nerve, and to explore the influence of this nerve on the brain and the body in general, they came up with electrical stimulation devices to stimulate the vagus nerve. The stimulation of this nerve by means of electrical energy is popularly referred to as vagus nerve stimulation (VNS), which has been proven to help treat people with epilepsy and treatment-resistant depression.

Vagus nerve stimulation is a medical treatment, and part of an increasingly popular field called bioelectronics which through the vagus nerve, makes use of tested clinically devices (surgically implanted on the chest wall with a wire running from it to the vagus nerve in the neck) to hack the body's nervous system by sending mild pulses of electrical energy to the brain. Depending on the specific needs of the patient, these mild pulses are sent at periodic intervals all through the day at an individualized dosage level of frequency and amplitude.

In 1997, the FDA approved the use of an implantable (and invasive) VNS to reduce the severity of epileptic seizures in epileptic patients that were unresponsive to medications. According to the Epilepsy Foundation, when VNS was administered to epileptic patients, it provided periodic stimulation to the vagus nerve, which in turn decreased, and or in rare cases, stopped the brain activity that caused the seizures. Researchers began noticing a range of unexpected but positive side effects in the administration of the VNS treatments to patients. For example, it was noticed that patients who had a reduction in epileptic seizures after being administered the VNS treatment also had a noticeable improvement in their moods. Not only that, but symptoms of depression became fewer, systemic inflammation lowered, and severe headaches were reportedly reduced. Officially in 2002, the initial observations made by researchers on how VNS aborted migraine headaches in patients with epilepsy were published in the paper, thereby giving rise to the possibility of using VNS in the treatment of migraine headaches.

In 2005, the FDA also approved the use of an implantable VNS to treat people with treatment-resistant depression and has also been found helpful in treating conditions such as bipolar disorder, anxiety disorders, and Alzheimer's disease.

Further medical applications in the use of VNS were reported. A study published in the Proceedings of the National Academy of Sciences (PNAS) in 2016, showed that vagus nerve stimulation using a bioelectronic device improved the condition of patients with rheumatoid arthritis, an inflammatory disease that is reported to have affected 1.3 million people in the US and costing billions of dollars to treat annually.

Surgically implanting a VNS device comes with some risks, some of which include difficulty swallowing, vocal cord paralysis, hoarseness, throat pain, headaches, cough, shortness of breath, prickling of the skin, and insomnia to mention but a few. Most people can tolerate these side effects and may lessen with time, but for but some people, the side effects could be bothersome in as much as the VNS device is implanted. Adjusting the electrical impulses is a great way to reduce these side effects. However, if they remain intolerable, the device can be shut down temporarily or permanently. Luckily, with the advancement of technology, other devices for electrical stimulation that are neither invasive nor require implantation have been developed and approved to serve certain types of conditions. In view of this, the FDA approved the use of the transcutaneous VNS device called gammaCore, for the treatment of migraines and cluster headaches in the US, which has also been cleared for use in Europe. The gammaCore is a hand-held VNS device that is administered by gently pressing the device against the neck to stimulate the vagus nerve. Another transcutaneous VNS device is the NEMOS system, a device which when applied to the ear, stimulates the vagus nerve. At this time, it has been cleared in the treatment of epilepsy and depression in Europe.

The use of VNS devices does not come cheap, which is why following through with the natural exercises and practices, food and diet supplements or other non-electrical passive methods earlier discussed would be a great way to activate your vagus nerve and still address the health conditions associated with the vagus nerve. Whatever treatment method you decide to use or if you decide to combine several methods (depending on your specific health issue), they are all effective means through which you can improve your health from conditions such as chronic inflammation, anxiety, depression, and epilepsy among others.

Conclusion

I'd like to thank you and congratulate you for transiting my lines from start to finish.

I hope this book was able to help you understand the different health conditions that can arise when your vagus nerve is damaged, and why it is very important that you be mindful of your lifestyle habits as well as the food and substances you allow into your body. And most importantly, I hope that you found the methods of vagus stimulation shared in this book to be quite useful to help you get started in stimulating your vagus nerve and taking charge of your health and wellbeing for good.

At this point, you are now better equipped to take control of your health. The next step is to apply your preferred method of stimulation, be it the active exercises and practice, passive methods, or even the food and diet supplement tips that I discussed in the previous chapter of this book. This book has shown you the unlimited potentials that you can unlock for your health when you stimulate your vagus nerve. So, I urge you to feel free to experiment which of these methods would work best for your needs and current health situation. Personally, increasing my vagal tone through the stimulation of my vagus nerve afforded me the ability to overcome anxiety and depression, and some other conditions I once suffered from. This has also helped me better manage similar conditions when they arise.

Finally, I want you to take personal responsibility for your health and wellbeing by incorporating the tips I have shared in this book into your daily life routine. As you regularly follow through with your preferred exercise and practice, tip or method, the more likely your vagus nerve becomes stimulated.

Remember…

"Knowing is not enough; we must apply. Willing is not enough; we must do" –Goethe.

I wish you the very best on your journey toward health and wellness!

References

The Vagus Nerve (CN X) - Course - Functions - TeachMeAnatomy. (2019, January 28). Retrieved from https://teachmeanatomy.info/head/cranial-nerves/vagus-nerve-cn-x/

Kenhub. (2020, February 27). Vagus nerve. Retrieved from https://www.kenhub.com/en/library/anatomy/the-vagus-nerve

Seymour, T. (2017, June 28). Everything you need to know about the vagus nerve. Retrieved from https://www.medicalnewstoday.com/articles/318128#What-is-the-vagus-nerve

9 Fascinating Facts About the Vagus Nerve. (2018, November 13). Retrieved from https://www.mentalfloss.com/article/65710/9-nervy-facts-about-vagus-nerve

Jayne, P. (2019, September 19). Penelope Jayne. Retrieved from https://www.globalrecharge.guru/vagus-nerve-the-body-mind-connection/

Leonard, J. (2019, May 28). 10 ways to improve gut health. Retrieved from https://www.medicalnewstoday.com/articles/325293

Dukovac, N. (2019, September 27). Vagal Nerve Tone, Heart Rate Variability and Chiropractic. Retrieved from https://www.adelaidefamilychiro.com/blog/vagal-tone-heart-rate-variability-and-chiropractic

Validation of the Apple Watch for Heart Rate Variability Measurements during Relax and Mental Stress in Healthy Subjects. (2018, August 1). Retrieved from https://www.ncbi.nlm.nih.gov/pmc/articles/PMC6111985/

Hack Your Vagus Nerve to Feel Better: 14 Easy Ways. (2019, August 12). Retrieved from https://victoriaalbina.com/vagusnerve/

Holland, K. (2019, April 18). Mercury Detox: Separating Fact from Fiction. Retrieved from https://www.healthline.com/health/mercury-detox#reducing-exposure

Harvard Health Publishing. (2019, November 5). The sweet danger of sugar. Retrieved from https://www.health.harvard.edu/heart-health/the-sweet-danger-of-sugar

GÁL, K. (2020, January 20). What are the best sources of omega-3? Retrieved from https://www.medicalnewstoday.com/articles/323144#omega-3-supplements

Harvard Health Publishing. (2019, November 5). The sweet danger of sugar. Retrieved from https://www.health.harvard.edu/heart-health/the-sweet-danger-of-sugar

Zope, S. A., & Zope, R. A. (2013, January). Sudarshan kriya yoga: Breathing for health. Retrieved from https://www.ncbi.nlm.nih.gov/pmc/articles/PMC3573542/#:~:text=Neurophysiological model of vagus nerve stimulation pathways&text=To summarize, improved autonomic function, amygdala, and stria terminalis.

The Vagus Nerve and the Healing Promise of The Sudarshan Kriya. (n.d.). Retrieved from https://www.artofliving.org/us-en/the-vagus-nerve-and-the-healing-promise-of-Sudarshan-Kriya

Harvard Health Publishing. (n.d.). The gut-brain connection. Retrieved from https://www.health.harvard.edu/diseases-and-conditions/the-gut-brain-connection

Levac, K. A. (n.d.). Research on Diaphragmatic Breathing. Retrieved from https://www.nqa.org/index.php?option=com_dailyplanetblog&view=entry&year=2019&month=07&day=01&id=35:research-on-diaphragmatic-breathing

www.ingramcontent.com/pod-product-compliance
Lightning Source LLC
Chambersburg PA
CBHW071711020426
42333CB00017B/2228